The Truth about Premature Ejaculation and Natural Solutions to Lasting Longer in Bed. . .

Nick Stanton

Published by:
Nick Stanton and Random Technologies
4409 HOFFNER AVENUE, SUITE 347
Belle Isle, FL 32812
Website: **http://www.MensGrowth.com**

Disclaimer

This book is intended as a reference material, not as a medical manual to replace the advice of your physician or to substitute for any treatment prescribed by your physician.

If you are ill or suspect that you have a medical problem, we strongly encourage you to consult your medical, health, or other competent professional before adopting any of the suggestions in this book or drawing inferences from it. If you are taking prescription medication, you should never change your diet (for better or worse) without consulting your physician, as any dietary change may affect the metabolism of that prescription drug.

This book and the author's opinions are solely for informational and educational purposes.

Individual results may vary.

Table of Contents

Abstract

Congratulations on taking the first step to treating premature ejaculation.

Premature ejaculation is a difficult condition and can have grave effects on the psychological wellbeing of the impacted individual. The good news is that thousands of men have overcome their premature ejaculation woes with a series of techniques and exercises that deliver a permanent solution to the problem.

Unlike many of the products and books on the market to counteract the problem, this report offers solutions that address the issue rather than hide the issue. While this may mean that any improvements will not be seen immediately, it does mean the problems causes will be steadily enhanced.

As each individual responds differently to the various exercises and techniques contained in this document, the results could vary, but we expect the majority of subjects could achieve satisfactory results in 1-12 weeks.

As each day passes, it is expected that your lasting power will improve.

Undoubtedly, the news that premature ejaculation is curable will be exciting to you. This report should be considered the complete guide to finding ways to manage your ejaculations, as we touch on the wide range of contributing factors and the methods involving the mental state, the physical body factors, physiological factors, and communicative strategies to manage the problem.

Please take your time to familiarize yourself with the contents of this report. In its entirety the information continued herein is expected to get you performing better in bed, and leading to a happier you and a more meaningful sexual relationship.

Thanks for reading.

Overview

Premature Ejaculation is not an issue that is unique to you.

In fact, over half of all men will experience it at some point in their lives. That doesn't mean that they are bad at sex, it does not mean that their partner is not satisfied sexually, and it doesn't make you inferior than the rest of the population.

While it can be psychologically damaging and frustrating, it doesn't have to be. In the majority of cases, men can improve their sexual duration by performing a host of exercises and trying visualization and mind tricks to get closer to their ideals of sexual gratification.

Based purely on numbers, the chances are that some of your friends and colleagues also suffer from a lack of stamina. But the reality is, there is no such thing as a 'sexual stud' and premature ejaculation does not warrant beating yourself up each night over your sex lives.

In addition with equipping you with the tools to fight the demons, the purpose of this report is to put the problem in perspective and explain how common it is. You're not alone. Nor are you alone in wanting to tackle premature ejaculation. That is why we've developed a series of exercises, breathing exercises, sexual positions and more that will result in the sexual performance you've always wanted.

Positivity and motivation will be the keys to reducing the chances of premature ejaculation on an immediate and sustained basis. Trust us and join us on a journey to self-improvement and gratification by reading and embracing the contents of this carefully prepared report.

We look forward to sharing in your success and improving your state of mind in relation to premature ejaculation.

Introduction on Arousal

Listening To Your Body

It is widely suggested that the majority of men are not entirely educated when it comes to sex and arousal. Very few think about sex from a critical body function and never fully understand how their bodies interact and respond to sex.

We suspect most men understand little more than the act of sex and the act of ejaculation, without ever learning the intricacies of arousal and mastering the management of the different stages of arousal. That is not all that surprising given we're not given the opportunity to do so, instead we rely on pornography.

Whether you've never had sex before or been having sex for thirty years, this report will give you the opportunity to understand your body and understand how to control your climaxes. All it takes is teaching your mind and body to control the whole process.

It's very important that you become completely familiar with each separate stage of sexual excitement. You will also want to become familiar with everything you think and feel during the whole process. Once you establish how you are reacting in mind and body during sexual arousal, you will be one step closer to having ejaculation control.

When you are sexually aroused, there are many mental and physical reactions that begin to take place. As each of these reactions occurs, you are becoming more aroused, which in turn gets you closer and closer to having an orgasm. You will begin to experience the following:

- Increased heart rate
- Blood pressure increase
- Testicles draw closer to body
- Breathing increases rapidly
- Leg muscles tense up
- Butt muscles tense up
- Foot muscles often tense up
- Pelvic muscles tense up
- Strong sense of euphoria
- Difficulty focusing on outside world
- Difficulty thinking rationally

Knowing that your body and mind will respond in the ways listed above, you can now become aware of them as they occur. Try to familiarize yourself with your breathing, your thinking, and your physical reactions, which although trick at the start, will be an important phase of the awareness process.

Reacting to the sensations as they occur may mean that rather than breathing out of your mouth, you recognize the need to breathe out your nose, which has a natural calming affect and focuses your attention away from the arousal.

Likewise, and as strange as it may sound, if you're moving too slowly in anticipation of ejaculation, speed things up.

Basically, start to appreciate and understand your body and react to the different movements and thoughts to delay your orgasm. Becoming aware of your sexual persona will take time, but it's very, very powerful once you reach your level of comfort and heightened awareness.

Stages of Arousal

The exact number of stages of arousal is often debated. Some literature has the number at as low as two whereas others have suggest it might be as high as 10. This report will favor the notion that there are just five stages that cover the process from arousal to climax.

As we have already suggested, each of these stages will form a crucial role in the sexual encounters and ultimate orgasm of the individual and each stage therefore needs to be considered and practiced individually. The following chapter will give a brief description of each stage before recommending some exercises and techniques unique to each that will help you control your orgasms and end your premature ejaculation woes.

The stages of arousal are:

1. First an initial trigger sparks interest in a male. This trigger can be either physical or psychological. The male may not necessarily experience an erection at this stage, but there is a general feeling of being sexually 'turned on'.

2. Now that the arousal level has been raised, the erection is likely to follow. With that come the other functions associated with an erection, namely, an increased heart rate and increased blood flow. This is usually support by some intimacy like touching or kissing.

3. Following the initial touching and kissing is usually direct contact with the penis, which could mean either touching of the penis, oral sex or penetration. At this point the male

is getting even more aroused.

4. When all arousal reactions occur simultaneously, the heart rate and blood pressure continue to increase, the muscles tense up and the general feelings of euphoric is evident. With the blood flow to the penis and the heightened arousal, orgasm is close.

5. When the sexual pleasure and arousal reactions have reached their peaks, meaning the body and mind is doing everything it can to reach climax. The male reaches a point where climax is inevitable. Immediately after orgasm, the arousal reaction slow down and the penis becomes flaccid once more.

The stages above are not widely known amongst the majority of men, which makes premature ejaculation even more common. But having said that some men become aware of them sub-consciously or later in life through experience, for example thinking of distractions and the height of orgasm is a technique everyday males often opt for. Unfortunately, these stages don't have a set time frame and can all occur within two minutes.

To control your climaxes, it is crucial that you understand the stages above and try and relate them back to your current sexual activity. As you approach stage five, to delay ejaculation you must control your mind to remain in stage four for as long as possible, delivering intense pleasure without the orgasm. This will revolutionize your sex life and the pleasure you derive from sex.

The following sections of this report will teach you how to do so.

The Psychology behind Premature Ejaculation

Stress

A males inability to last during sex can wreak havoc on their psyche and sexual confidence, not only does this lead to stress, but stress can also be the cause of the premature ejaculations. The stress could be due to your feelings towards family, work, finances or health, and can affect you in ways beyond the root of the stress, often negatively.

Many experts believe that stress outside the bedroom lead to stress in the bedroom

As men we often bury and internalize our feelings (especially those that are considered week) so we don't have to deal with them or discuss the topic. This are of the brain is called the subconscious, but can still bring negativity to the surface in other ways.

If these stresses are not properly dealt with it will only make your premature ejaculation worse. It is therefore recommend approaching your stresses head on, so that you can work towards a clear head and an edifying sex life. The report aims to teach you ways to create harmony between your body and your mind. Without the techniques the external pressures can mean some males struggle to get an erection, experience premature ejaculation or avoid sex completely. Once these changes begin, it sets the wheels in motion for stress in every situation and deeper levels of despair.

This report focuses on premature ejaculation not stress relief, so although it's important to identify and control the stress in your life, this report can only ask you pinpoint where the stress is coming from it and remedy it. Then the report will show you how to be a better lover.

Despite that, some of the recommendations, exercises and techniques may work to help eliminate everyday stress. But don't wait to make changes to your life, take charge now.

Sexual Stress

Sexual stress is another source of frustration and another potential cause of premature ejaculation. It can be exclusive from everyday stress but still creates an intense pressure to preform sexually and satisfy their sexual partners.

Historically, men were focused almost entirely on spreading their seed and helping a community's population grow. Therefore they did so quickly and with scant regard to leisure. Sex performed quickly with a speedy ejaculation ensures the survival of a species and a bloodline.

But in this day and age, men think on a much higher level yet still suffer from premature ejaculation. Men are increasingly under pressure to perform due to the influence of the pornography industry, the way an orgasm is depicted in mainstream media and the younger age that people are having sex and becoming sexually aware and experimental. Accordingly, anxiety, stress, and nervousness begin to take hold and control the physical body, and it becomes impossible to control the body and its reactions.

When the mind is not alert (and distracted by social pressures) the body too cannot work at its best, making it impossible for the body to pick up the signals the mind is giving it and vice versa. This means that controlling the way your body reacts during the arousal phases becomes extremely tricky.

When your body is out of sync during sex, your stamina and lasting power suffer greatly.

Anxiety also fuels adrenaline, which when flowing through the body is similar to the heightened awareness and feelings an athlete might get before a big race. Athletes harness that energy and adrenalin, whereas in the bedroom it inhibits and more often than not results in a feeling many of us know all too well, premature ejaculation.

The good news once again, is that you need not worry. All of the techniques that are described in this report will benefit you in life and in sex.

Even those with a steady and mind and only rare premature ejaculation experiences will benefit from the mind and sexual tips contained herein.

Embracing the Negativity

Because our mind plays such an important role in all of our lives – including our sex lives, it is an important tool to train to behave the way in which you want it to (especially in the bedroom). Understandably, this creates a dramatically negative thought in the mind which impacts sexual performance and general self-esteem.

To counteract the negativity, this report suggests that bottling the energy, and using it to your favor can deliver some great sexual results. It only takes a simple switch in your thinking to something more positive to have your body function equally as positively and like a well-oiled machine. This positivity can be transferred to the bedroom, and also as seen in athletes, confidence can produce exceptional results.

Our simple techniques will teach you how to bring anxiety levels down to a more relaxed state that results in a much more relaxed state of mind and increased sexual composure levels. All in all resulting in a far greater sexual experience with delayed orgasm.

Exercise: Relaxation

Relaxation is a crucial ingredient to good sex. But this is often difficult to achieve given the impact of sexual arousal.

In order to practice our first relaxation technique, you'll need a comfortable spot with little noise and no distractions. Begin the exercise with a clear mind, and in an environment clear of clutter and electronic devices. Any distraction that is likely to break your concentration needs to be identified and removed from the environment.

Here's how the exercise works:

- Lie down where you feel very comfortable. This could be on the floor, couch, or bed. It's up to you. Obviously you know where you are most comfortable. If you need to, use a pillow to get even more comfortable.

- Close your eyes, and lie on your back with your arms to your side. If you want to, play some soothing music like quiet nature sounds such as waves, water or rain drops.

- Clear your mind of everything that is running through it each day. Work, school, study, bills, family, and so on.

Instead, focus on your breathing, counting each inhale as 1 and each exhale as 2. Breathe in through your nose and out through your mouth and hold each breathe for two seconds. Imagine all the air that you exhale running through your entire body. Become completely relaxed. You can also try and visualize a memory where you remember being extremely comfortable and relaxed. Focus on that memory.

- As you continue let yourself drift away, like you are falling asleep. After doing this for about 10 minutes, your mind should be relaxed. This state is known as deep relaxation.

Now that you are in a relaxed state, it is time to focus on your body. Continue the exercise in the same manner, but this time become aware of your body parts.

Start at the top with your head, ears, eyes, nose, and mouth. Slowly tense and then relax your arms, hands, bottom, genitals, thighs, calves, and feet – all individually. Start at the top of your body, and do each body part one at a time, working your way down to your feet and toes. There is no need to rush either. Take it slowly, focusing on each tension and relaxation of each body part.

What this does is teaches your body to be conscious of each of its individual parts. Further, it teaches you to control each body part deliberately. The results of which are, overtime, you will become completely in sync with each and every part of your body, which will help in some of the other exercises explained in this report.

Breathing

You're now ready to try this relaxation and breathing technique when you're having sex or masturbating. The next time you are masturbating or having sex, pay very close attention to your breathing. You'll notice that your breathing changes through each stage of the arousal process. At times it may quicken and at other times slow, at times you may be using your nose and at others breathing through your mouth.

It's good to be aware of these changes and if you're especially committed jot down the results to revert back to down the track. It's all part of the process of taking control of the factors affecting premature ejaculation and becoming more aware.

Our breathing can have a direct influence on the heart rate and the level of arousal. An example of this is during masturbation whereby most men take fast, short breaths during sex and masturbation. Concerning, this can cause over arousal.

Rather, we encourage taking slow and deep breaths at an interval of about 3-4 seconds. While difficult to grasp at the beginning it is important to try and keep this pace and keep the breathing consistent (e.g. through the nose or mouth but not both, same intervals and same thoughts).

Practice will bring greatly consistency and after a while you can expect to get much better at keeping a breathing rhythm.

Because your breathing an arousal levels are connected it also means your breathing and point of orgasm are also correlated. If they are connected it means, if you control one aspect, you're controlling both.

For example, you can pinpoint when you are going to get too excited, and slow down the process, without hindering you or your partner's pleasure. With this breathing technique it will in turn will allow you to last longer.

Knowing when you are breathing either incorrectly, too fast, or not breathing at all, allows you to make the necessary adjustments to slow it back down, breathe properly, decrease your anxiety level, and ultimately prolong the sexual intercourse you're engaged in.

Exercise: Breathing

Having explained the importance of the nose and mouth in breathing, it can also be said that even if the methods suggested earlier are used, anxiety can still eventuate and you will still ejaculate too quickly.

Therefore, breathing using the diaphragm is also important to achieving relaxation and longer lasting sex. It is important to expand the diaphragm and the lower ribs completely, but not your upper chest, when taking a proper deep breath. If you breathe through your upper body and chest, your breaths will become too constrained.

Try breathing from the diaphragm and feel the difference it makes to the depth of your breath. Experts believe that this method of breathing can result in more endurance during the day, and during sex. Breathing only from your chest takes away the energy from the diaphragm and won't deliver the breathing gains needed to control your orgasm.

An excellent exercise for this particular breathing is explained below, it can be used during sex or during masturbation.

Keep a nice steady pace of slow, deep breaths through the nose and out the mouth. Slowly close your eyes every 15-40 seconds and take in a very deep breath through your nose. When you have your eyes closed, you should be concentrating fully on every breath that you take. Become fully aware of everything involved with that breath. Try your best not to think about the sex or masturbation that is taking place. Think about your breathing only.

- Hold it for 5 seconds, and then let it out slowly. Like I said, repeat this every 15-40 seconds, depending on the severity level of your premature ejaculation. If you are aroused very, very quickly, you will want to do this frequently, maybe even more often than every 15 seconds. For those of you who can last for at least a little bit, you can do this less frequently.

Not only is this exercise easy but it's also highly effective. This helps you remain calm, and keeps arousal levels low while still being able to enjoy the excitement of a sexual encounter or masturbation.

Exercise: Breathing

Yet another breathing technique that is also very easy to follow and implement, but can also yield great results in delaying your ejaculation combines the practice of deep and relaxing breathing with the simulation of sex.

This exercise is best practiced during sex but it can work during masturbation too. It works by timing your inhales with your pull back motions and your exhales with your pump or penetration motions. Because we've explained the importance of slow and concentrated breathing you won't be able to do this during every motion but instead try with each 4-8 thrust motions. This will bring immediate improvements to your lasting power.

If you are trying this during masturbating, consider each downward stroke of your hand as a thrust into the vagina, and each upward stroke of your hand as a thrust pulling out of the vagina. So you will want to exhale when your hand is moving down and you will want to inhale when your hand is going up towards the head of your penis.

The retraining of your mind and the reinforcement of repeated movements and breathes aims to retrain your mind and body. This will become crucial to you in your sexual endeavors and in some of the lessons to be learned throughout this report. In doing so, you should notice that your anxiety and stress levels tail off and the pressure you were once under lifted.

Visualization

As with all tasks and experiences associated with life, having a positive attitude plays a major role in the success and enjoyment you have when completing the tasks. By removing the negative connotations and influence of the negative stigmas attached to premature ejaculation, you will find yourself enjoying sex more and be able to perform for longer. No matter how down you're feeling, stop, rid your mind of the negative and focus on the positive.

Try to reaffirm within yourself that you can take control of your stamina issues, you can last longer in bed, and you can delay orgasm for as long as you want. By repeating it, you will start to believe it, and as you believe it you're staying power will adjust, and your confidence will improve.

This method of positive reinforcement, works wonders when combined with visualization techniques. For instance, visualize yourself having amazing sex. You can even use the method to counter a specific bedroom or sexual problem. If it's a problematic position that is making you orgasm more quickly, visualize yourself having sex in that position for a long time, if you're too attracted to your partners appearance, start to visualize being with her (or other attractive females) more often.

To make the sensation even more real, you can walk through the entire experience, from meeting a girl, to dancing, to kissing, foreplay and sex. Go into detail, visualize what it would be like to be insider your partner, the smells, the tastes and sounds.

All the while making the experience enjoying and fulfilling. It is no goo to bring up more anxiety, so picture you doing everything right and start to picture the breathing techniques we talked about earlier. Start to think about how relaxed you are, how your breathing is under control, yet be impressed by how good the sex is.

This creates a benchmark that you believe you have hit in the past. In a way it tricks you're mind to believe it has actually happened and you can actually do it. To practice, do this on a daily basis, for 5-10 minutes, and you can expect actual bedroom results.

Many of the world's greatest minds and greatest athletes have appreciate the worth of visualization and just how effective the mind can be at harnessing energy and producing amazing accomplishments. With continued practice, you too, can reap the rewards of visualization practice.

The Physical Side of Premature Ejaculation

Rewire Your Body

It's not uncommon to blame someone, or something for your premature ejaculation. One of the major sources of blame and frustration is the body. A vast amount of men believe there is nothing they can do to make themselves last longer, they simply see it as a physical condition and don't believe that you can retrain your body with exercises and techniques (maybe due to the amount of spam emails on the topic).

However, in this section we explain just how improvements can be made and how each of you can rewire your body.

A strong example of teaching your body to adapt to a different exercise or movement is in the training of marathon runners. When they enter a marathon, they don't run a marathon the next day. They build up their fitness, stamina and mindset over time and based on a specific and gradual system. It is the same with weightlifters. They don't try and lift as much as they humanely can every single day.

Based on the above logic, and the experience of hundreds of men, the same can be said for sexual prowess. To get better, you need to work on certain physical attributes of your body that are involved with ejaculation. If you do, there's no reason why your muscles won't strengthen and develop, and there's no reason why you can't enjoy better sex.

As you're reading you're hopefully beginning to understand

the potential to conquer your condition, with a combination of physical and psychological methods.

PC Muscle

The PC muscle (pubococcgeus muscle) is found in both men and women, and stretches from the coccyx (tail bone) to the pubic bone, and is just one of a group of muscles that form the pelvic floor. This muscle cradles the internal sexual genitalia.

The PC muscle is involved in urine control and flow, and is the muscle responsible for allowing men to move their penis up and down when it is erect. It is also the muscle used for holding back bowel movements. More importantly, however, it is involved in the orgasm process. A well-developed PC muscle can enhance the sexual experience in both men and women, and that includes the orgasm as well.

The easiest way to find your PC muscles is to actually feel it working. The next time you go to the bathroom, try and stop your urination in mid-stream. Or, you can try to push out those last few dribbles. The muscle that is controlling that is your PC muscle. You can immediately determine if you have a lot of control or very little control just by testing it during urination.

You can also flex your erect penis up and down. You can actually feel muscles squeeze at the base of your penis. Those are your PC muscles. If you can't flex it 25 times in a row, or hold it flexed for 20 seconds, you have an underdeveloped muscle.

For interests sake, you should try and locate your PC muscle now, and because it is involved in the ejaculatory process, you should take the time to understand its movements and your control of those movements, as it will have a big impact on your staying power.

Very few men understand and comprehend how to use this muscle, which is mainly due to the lack of education around the muscle. Simply put, we've never been taught how to use it or been given a reason to try and strengthen it.

A weak PC muscle, can lead to:

1. Having trouble detecting your arousal level during the 5 stages of arousal. This leads to overexcitement, and inevitably premature ejaculation.

2. Weak ejaculations, that have very little force and consistency.

3. Having difficulty sustaining and maintaining a full erection.

4. Having to wait a long time between ejaculations and sex sessions, before being ready for action again.

Having said that, there are ways to strengthen it and prevent the possibilities listed above from occurring. The strengthening exercises that this report will go into will lead you towards fuller, stronger ejaculations, as well as a greater understanding of your place in the arousal process during sex.

Some students have lasted as much as 10 minutes longer in bed in less than a week making a strong PC muscle one of the key pillars of a healthy sex life.

Exercise: PC Muscle

As with a lot of the exercises this report teaches you (aside from the sex and masturbation exercises), the PC muscle improvement technique can be done anywhere. You don't necessarily need to be naked or even able to see your penis. We simply suggest you're comfortable and ready to concentrate.

It's important to do these exercises at your own pace, just like the exercise example above, you don't need to overexert yourself right from the get go. Keep building and you should see vast improvements. The following exercises are called Kegel exercises. Kegels are designed to strengthen and give voluntary control over the PC muscle. They are named after the doctor who invented them, Dr. Arnold Kegel.

Here's how they work (it is recommended you do these with 'semi' erection at about 50% of its full capabilities):

PC Muscle Exercises

1. Quickly flex the muscle by squeezing and releasing it. (By now you should have an idea of how to "flex" or "squeeze" the muscle). You are not actually using your hands to squeeze it. The squeezing is the contraction of the muscle. Squeeze and hold for 1-2 seconds, and then release. Rest for 1-2 seconds, and then repeat the process.

You should do this 20 times, 3-4 times a week, during week 1. The following chart shows the progression of the exercise. Please note that you can increase and do more reps each week if you feel comfortable. Starting with 20 is just a frame of reference to see where you stand. However, do not move on to the next week until you can complete 60 reps in each stage.

So, if you can only do 40 flexes in week 1, 3-4 days a week, then do not move on to week 2 until you can do 60 flexes. Once you can hold the flex for the appropriate amount of time 60 different times, 3-4 days a week (every other day basically), then you can move on to the next week.

Weekly Progression of Exercise 1

Week	Reps	Time Holding Squeeze	Rest between Reps
1	20-60	1-2 seconds	1-2 seconds
2	20-60	3-4 seconds	3-4 seconds
3	25-60	6-8 seconds	5-6 seconds
4	30-60	10-12 seconds	5-6 seconds
5	30-60	15-20 seconds	6-10 seconds

Be aware of your breathing during these exercises and try and keep a consistent and rhythmic breathing pattern. This is achieved by exhaling when you contract the PC muscle and inhaling when you're relaxing. These measures will make it more beneficial in the long term.

2. This exercise is similar to the first exercise, but with a couple of key differences. Start by flexing the PC muscle very slowly, not quickly like you did in exercise 1. Once fully flexed, it should take 3-5 seconds before you can relax and inhale.

In order to ensure you're performing the exercise correctly, monitor the reaction of your anus and testicles. They should tingle, which is a sign that you are indeed strengthening your PC muscle.

The chart below sets out an exercise regime for this particular exercise and gives an indication of the length of time you should be holding the pulse for and then how long you should be relaxing for:

Weekly Progression of Exercise 2

Week	Reps	Time Holding Squeeze	Rest between Reps
1	10-30	1-2 seconds	1-2 seconds
2	10-30	3-4 seconds	3-4 seconds
3	15-30	6-7 seconds	5-6 seconds
4	15-30	8-10 seconds	5-6 seconds
5	20-30	10-12 seconds	6-10 seconds

3. The third Kegel exercise is a recreation of the feeling you experience when you need to move your bowels, except you obviously will not be going to the bathroom this time. To try this at home, push down through your lower stomach, as if you were passing urine. Do not tense your stomach too much and try to focus pushing with your PC muscle instead. Complete

5-15 reps, for 5-15 seconds, with rests of 3-15 seconds in between at your own pace.

Here's a weekly schedule which will help you balance the three different exercises. The exercises are listed as 1, 2, and 3, and correspond to the 3 exercises mentioned above.

Weekly Schedule for PC Muscle Exercises

Monday	Tuesday	Wednesday	Thursday	Friday	Saturday	Sunday
1	2, 3	1	23	1	23	1

Progression should be evident from week to week and if you follow the exercise regime in addition to the breathing and relaxation strategies there should be noticeable differences in the length of time you can make love for.

Multiple Orgasms for Men

It is possible to have an orgasm without ejaculating. Multiple orgasms in men are similar to the experience that women feel when they climax on multiple occasions. Although difficult to master, it essentially involves getting close to orgasm without actually ejaculation and holding it for some time. The feeling is described as intense and deeply satisfying.

Ultimately, the successful performance of this technique comes down to resisting the urge to ejaculate. To practice, in masturbation or intercourse, tightly flex your PC muscle for 2-6 seconds before you feel like climaxing. Keep doing so until the urge has passed.

This goes against all our natural instincts, and accordingly, will be very hard to learn, but once you've mastered it you should be able try it multiple times during one sex session without losing an erection.

Many authors in the area only suggest trying this technique when you are already adept at controlling your PC muscle and the other breathing techniques already mentioned.

Masturbation Training for Lasting Longer

Masturbation is a great way to practice real sexual techniques including when trying to improve your stamina. We usually masturbate quickly, but in order to master masturbation for the purposes of lasting longer in bed you'll need to practice doing so in a more relaxed state.

Masturbate with a woman's orgasm in mind, not your own. In other words, take your time. You should masturbate when you've got 10 to 20 minutes spare to dedicate to it. Experiment with different techniques to truly master your lasting ability. One such practice technique could be to bring yourself close to the point of no return, but don't let yourself ejaculate until time is up.

Masturbation is one of the best ways to understand how your body responds to sex in order to train yourself to last longer in bed. However, not all masturbation will help you and in fact it can train you to orgasm faster if done incorrectly.

Here's how to use masturbation to improve your ability to delay your orgasm:

- First and foremost, always us a lubricant. What this does is simulate the feeling of the vagina and recreates the actual feeling of penetration more than the sensitivity of a dry hand. This is all part of the recreation and visualization of the experience, and because the feeling of masturbation with a lubricant is so good, it lowers the sensitivity levels during intercourse.

- Secondly, remember to breathe correctly – in line with the methods we alluded to earlier.

- As always be aware of your arousal level. If you feel your ejaculation is coming on, slow down or take a quick break.

Exercise: Masturbation: 1 Second Stroke

Although some research on training masturbation will have you masturbate without visualization or stimulation, we favor an approach that stimulates sex as closely as possible. While we all have different aids that help us get aroused, it could be pornographic videos, erotic pictures, or strong memory of a past encounter. Whatever it is, for this exercise you'll need it handy and you'll need to be aroused. You'll also need at least 15 minutes and you'll need lubricant too.

Begin in a position that stimulates the most. That could be lying on your back, sitting in a chair, imitating doggy style or even standing up.

Now, once you are in your most stimulating position, erect and have applied the lube, begin to slowly masturbate. Keep a controlled and stead back and forth motion despite your level of arousal or the speed of which your visualization or pornographic aid is moving at. If you feel the urge to masturbate quicker, do not do it, concentrate on each stroke of your hand and visualize actual intercourse.

The point of this exercise is to continue masturbating even when you feel like you are going to ejaculate. Stop 20 seconds before the point of no return (which will become easier and easier as you try this method more and more).

Whether you ejaculate within seconds, minutes or hours or initiating sex, these techniques will work for you and allow you to control your orgasm. It may seem tedious or unnecessary if you fall in the longer categories above, but regardless of your situation you can have more fulfilling sex by practicing these methods.

Exercise: Masturbation: Quick Draw Method

The quick draw method is exactly as above but with a quicker movement, usually a few strokes per second. The 20-second rule still applies here, but the 20 seconds will come on quicker when working at a quicker pace.

Try not to cut corners, try not to lose interest and above all try not to climax.

Try to concentrate, try to visualize and try to take it seriously.

Practice makes perfect, especially with the quick draw method of intense masturbation. If the exercises are challenging for you at first, don't worry, it might take a bit longer to master than some of the other skills you've tried to pick up in the past, but to reassure you, you're on the right path and our techniques work.

Exercise: Masturbation: Combination Method

As the title of the exercise suggests, this method looks to combine the two exercises you learned above. The influence the individual exercise has is minimal, so you can start with whichever you prefer and alternate when you prefer.

All other things being equal, this third technique is reinforcing the habits you created by trying the two methods in isolation. This is because in intercourse the speed at which you're penis is stimulated varies depending on your speed and your partners.

To reiterate, practice correct masturbation by taking your time, because you don't want to finish until your woman does, so masturbate with that in mind. Set a time to work up to, something like 15 minutes and when you get close to finishing slow down, don't finish until time is up. This is one way to help train your body and your mind to **last longer in bed**.

Practice this technique, like the others, upwards of three times a week, and swap the exercises around to keep the regime interesting and to cover all your bases.

The Physiological Side of Premature Ejaculation

Healthy Living

The following section of this report will feature some reasoning behind the importance of healthy and balanced living, and how this can create a healthy sex life. Maintaining peak physical fitness can do wonders for premature ejaculation as evidenced in a number of reported studies, and the good news is you don't have to spend hours in a gym each week. As most professionals would prescribe for healthy living, we suggest just a couple of days a week of light weight lifting and cardio to improve your energy and sex life.

Equally as important is the diet and supplement system you adhere to in your everyday life. What we put into our bodies is crucial in your libido levels and overall wellness.

While there may be some pharmaceutical advancements (like Viagra) on the market that can assist with a variety of sexual related issues, it does not work for premature ejaculation. In fact, it has the opposite effect as most users experience heightened arousal leading to quicker climax. Therefore, it's important to fill your body with the type of materials and fuels that provide important nutrients for your body, that will allow you to relax more during sex, be more confident, and ultimately last longer before you reach orgasm.

Natural foods to increase testosterone and serotonin levels in your body can be purchased easily and have a big impact on the overall levels of the balance of the body.

Foods for Sexual Health

There are two major areas where your diet can affect your sexual lasting power. The first of which is Breakfast. As you are aware, breakfast is often described as the most important meal of the day as it delivers the energy for rest of the day. That includes sexual energy too. The best foods for prolonged energy and focus are:

- Foods that are high in riboflavin and thiamine can help you store energy more efficiently. If you are eating cereals and breads at breakfast.

- Foods that have a high level of niacin in them. Niacin allows histamine to flow in your body, which is important for delaying ejaculation.

The second major area where food groups can improve your sexual performance is connected with your circulation. Studies have shown that foods rich in L-Arginine such as peanuts, walnuts, cashews, dairy, oatmeal, granola, garlic, green vegetables, ginseng, root vegetables, seeds, soybeans, can improve sexual functionality in men by improving circulation.

Other foods known to help with the circulatory system are foods that are high in Omega-3 fatty acids. Salmon, mackerel, flaxseeds, halibut, and snapper are excellent sources for this nutrient. Omega-3 fatty acids also get your nervous system functioning better, which in turn helps with sexual health, depression, and fatigue.

Natural Supplementation with P.E.

Because premature ejaculation is often linked to depression and anxiety, some men believe they lack serotonin and that this causes their issues, whereas doctors may prescribe anti-depressants (such as Prozac) to suppress the negativity in the mind of the affected male.

While the anti-depressants can work for those that are severely depressed, for most of us it is unnecessary and can have side effects such as problems achieving an erection.

Therefore this report does not endorse any medication (natural or otherwise) to help with premature ejaculation.

Research continues to be conducted to find the magic cure or pill that will reduce the known cases of premature ejaculation (and it's likely to be a profitable search too), but in the meantime sign up to www.MensGrowth.com to receive alerts to our discoveries on this subject.

The boost is a way of replenishing muscles to their normal state and much like a bodybuilder would take supplements, this boost product can be used to gain extra staying power.

Sexual Positions and Techniques for Lasting Longer In Bed

Sex

At the end of the day, premature ejaculation relates to sex. We can teach you all the best known breathing, relaxation and masturbation techniques to improve your stamina but what you really want to know is how this will relate to improved bedroom performance. You might be thinking 'what if I follow your instructions to a t' and then still struggle in the bedroom.

In this section we explore ways to make you last longer during sex, with advice on sexual positions and ejaculatory control.

Sexual Positions

It is very evident when you're in the middle of intercourse that certain positions have different effects on your ability to hold off ejaculation. Just as different positions can offer different levels of pleasure, they can also deliver different levels of sensitivity to the man. The report will now give a rundown of the most common sexual positions and explain the best ways to improve stamina when engaged in each position.

Man on Top (Missionary)

The most common sexual position. The missionary position is the most widely used and probably the first position we all tried. It's easy and pleasurable for both parties.

Most experts believe that this position makes it difficult to control arousal but our research and experience suggests otherwise. Although the strain on the arms and legs is significant in this position, making it harder to support your body weight and ejaculation, the position is romantic and classical and at the very least the man controls the rate of penetration.

Missionary is the most intimate position as well. Couples can kiss and hug, staring into each other's eyes and watching facial expressions. It provides great stimulation for the clitoris and g-spot. If you try popping yourself up on your arms, raising your groin up a few inches, there will be increased stimulation through the contact of your pubic bone and the woman's vulva.

Try having her bend her legs, which will allow herself to open, and in turn will allow you to penetrate deeper. Your partner can put her feet under her hips and rise up with her pelvis in order to have better leverage and control. Another great technique is to use your butt for leverage.

Your partner places her hands on your butt, and pulls herself up to meet your strokes. She has control of the intensity of the position, varying rhythm and angle of pressure so she can maximize clitoral stimulation.

Also, try having her hold her legs together, while you position your legs on either side of hers. This will move the penis back and forth over the clitoris while you are penetrating her. This greatly increases pleasure for both partners.

Woman on Top

The second most popular sexual position is when the woman is on top. This can be done either with your partner facing you or with her back to you.

As a position it is so widely well received because the girl can control the sex speed and direction and in the same vein her own pleasure. It's often easier for the men to control their ejaculation.

Because you're on your back and in a relaxed state, it means you can pay closer attention to your stages of arousal, concentrate on your breathing, and engage your PC muscles. The renewed focus will allow you to become aware of your speed and motion and longer lasting sex.

Slight alterations to your positions can often times make a great difference, depending on what you want to achieve. Going faster, slower, moving hips or legs a bit, or bending in different ways can all achieve varying results.

Experiment with these no matter what you're trying to achieve, and while you're looking to better yourself in the stamina department you cannot be selfish, and you must try your hardest to make the experience enjoyable for you both.

Doggy Style

Doggy style is a position that is synonymous with animalism and instinct and delivers maximum excitement and appeal for men and women. For men, it's a feeling of dominance and for women the feeling is that they are being 'taken'. The position also leads itself to deep penetration and g-spot stimulation.

We recommend easing the pressure on your legs by avoiding

squatting, and instead, sitting on your knees, or standing at the edge of the bed.

In terms of orgasm control, when a woman is on her knees and pushes her backside up for doggy style, her body naturally opens up a bit more. This allows for deeper penetration, and less stimulation on the head of the penis, which will help you last longer.

A more intimate alternative doggy style experience can be having your partner lie flat on her stomach and you lying on top of her.   This allows for more intimate contact both physically and verbally.

Side by Side

Also known as spooning, this is a great position for lasting longer before orgasm. Not only that it also helps when you're tired, when you're up for morning sex, and if you have back problems or other physical limitations. Intimacy is again at its highest in this position with heavy kissing and hugging common.

It is best to "scissor" or intertwine your legs with your partners, instead of having her legs wrapped around you, this helps shift the weight and create a slightly new angle and position, which is good for control.

Standing

A slightly more risqué and less traditional position is standing up. If the moment takes you, the beauty of this position is that you can perform it anywhere that is safe. It can however be difficult due to height differences and angles.

Therefore, try with a prop such as a table or a wall, and experiment with angles and leg positions until you find something that is suitable for both and allows you to focus on controlling your arousal and subsequent ejaculation.

Delaying Your Orgasm

Even though the techniques already discussed in this report will have you on the right track to increased sexual staying power, there are still some techniques that you can use in the bedroom to delay orgasm while you are still in the ongoing training phase.

The first option is to where a condom every time you have sex. Not only is this safer for obvious reasons but it also desensitizes your penis and lengthen sex. They're easy to find and will have you increasing the duration of your sexual encounters.

Secondly, find a position that works for you. The report has described the most common positions that we all use, and one that works for one individual may not work for another. Accordingly, we suggest finding something that works to your individual and unique set of circumstance. Start with it and stick with it.

Looking back to the masturbation techniques we practiced earlier, if you found it easier to last longer with the slower method, then recreate that in the bedroom and vice versa for the quick draw method. Likewise, just before you reach orgasm pull out and slow down your thrusts.

Always remember to keep your breathing under control, and use the methods that were discussed in the breathing section of this book. You should also apply the PC muscle techniques as well.

If your partner is up for it, try breaking up the intensity of the sex with a normal conversation. This distraction method hopes to take away the urge to ejaculate and keeps the mind occupied on things other than arousal.

Another technique that you can try to counteract your premature ejaculations is to control your thrusts when you think you're near to ejaculating, by becoming aware of when you're close you can shorten your thrusts or enter your partner fully without thrusting to allow your arousal levels to drop.

When you are having sex, you are generally doing the in and out motion in missionary or doggy, and she is going up and down when she is on top. When you start realizing that your arousal level is getting higher, stop the thrusting motion. Remember, this should be well before you actually think you are going to have an orgasm.

So, you can constantly go back and forth. Thrust a few, then rest inside with little or no motion. Thrust again, then rest. The deeper you stay during sex, the less stimulation you will have. Many women get more pleasure having sex like this anyway.

Changing positions frequently can also help. This is because the constant movement and down time lowers the arousal level. Positively, women won't mind this as it keeps things exciting and gives off the impression that you're confident and dominant. This includes changing from intercourse to oral sex to rejuvenate you without the women losing her arousal.

There are also ways of completely stopping sex, getting re-charged, and then having sex again.

Now, when you put it all together, you can combine every one of these techniques. For example, you can start on bottom and have a normal conversation. Then tease, start foreplay and control your thrusts during intercourse in a teasing manner.

If you are give off and air of confidence that tells her you are in complete control, then she is going to love it. All of these techniques will send this message. And, with time, you will get better and better at lasting in different positions using different techniques. Soon you won't need the techniques and tips, and long lasting sex will become second nature.

The Importance of Communication

Men are from Mars and Women are from Venus is a well-known quote that describes the intricacies of men and women and how they communicate. Men tend to love physicality, whereas women love with more heart and more emotion. But sex is sex, no matter what gender.

Sometimes sex is good. Sometimes sex is bad. Sometimes sex is fast, and sometimes it's slow. It's never really the same with anyone. It's not worth worrying over as much as people do. This section will look at other ways to enjoy a fulfilling relationship, with communication and less emphasis on sex.

The Role of Pornography

Pornography damages our sex lives, but to what extent, experts often argue over. Some believe that porn is a terrible guideline for sex due to the unrealistic nature of it, the fact that the actors are professionals, the filming has been edited and the films are often catered to men not women. It makes se mechanical and robotic and lacking in intimacy. By relying on sex as a stimulant it teaches and trains you into bad habits that may affect your sex live and copy bad habits (quick movements) that could impact on your climax. Sex based on a porn script also lacks the emotional aspect often caved by the women (from Venus).

However, in the same way, porn trains our brains to release more endorphins than is natural in response to an overload of sexual stimuli. After a while, our brains become desensitized and develop a need for higher and higher stimuli in order to reach the same arousal and excitement. Thus begins the spiral into more hardcore porn and higher quantities of it.

Communicating Based on the Differences

It can sometimes feel that men and women are from different planets (hence the quote above), communication can be difficult between the two, which can cause frictions in relationships, and lingering problems.

Rest assured, there are a host of things men can do to make the communication process a whole lot easier. They are quite simple really, and will make a world of difference for you and your relationship.

In much the same way as becoming aware of premature ejaculation, you need to become aware of the differences that exist between men and women. You need to be clear that these will always be here, you need to be empathetic and you need to adjust to the differences. Specifically to sex, if a woman doesn't feel that she's being heard, she will start to freeze up emotionally, and sexually. This pattern will continue unless you break it.

Frustration like this can lead to frustration in the bedroom or a complete lack of willingness to partake in intimacy that most relationships crave.

So the answer is simple. Just listen. Regardless of what a woman wants to talk to you about, whether it's a story, emotional issue, concern, question, anything - she just wants you to listen. As previously alluded to, women seek an emotional connection, and one way to do that is by listening and communicating effectively.

Good communication is a fundamental part of a healthy relationship. When people stop communicating well, they stop relating well, and times of change or stress can really bring out disconnect. As long as you are communicating, you can work through whatever problem you're facing.

Honest, direct communication is a key part of any relationship. When both people feel comfortable expressing their needs, fears, and desires, trust and bonds are strengthened.

Furthermore, relationships deteriorate when what is needed and wanted is not expressed; the resulting frustrations build up and result in increasing anxiety and upset. This is particularly likely to occur with sexual relationships, when problems or disagreements about sexual issues are not discussed openly and honestly. If this is the case in your personal life, then here's how to go about improving matters. Note, this is an exercise to do with your sexual partner.

Foreplay vs. Sex

The advice about communication that we've listed above will hopefully strengthen your relationships and strengthen your sex life. That's important in building trust and developing a relationship that could eventuate in sex. It's important through communication that you get a women in the mood for sex.

Once she is, you can start to experiment within the realms of foreplay.

Keeping with the sports theme, men tend to warm up quickly

and then go out and play the game with little preparation. It may be an arrogant response which signals that we don't need the practice and are ready to perform from the outset.

But foreplay cannot follow the same blueprint. Guys tend to rush through foreplay and get stuck straight into sex. Not only is this disappointing for the women it also hints at a little bit of selfishness or lack of respect. But for those of us struggling with premature ejaculation, this actually plays into our hands. Essentially, because those suffering from stamina issues place increased importance on foreplay (usually to delay ejaculation) it means they're often held in higher esteem than men that rush foreplay.

Foreplay to women is more important than the sex, and foreplay for her begins with your overall communication with her. You must work on a women's brain before you work on her body. Seducing and relaxing her mind, then seducing and relaxing her body, will make her think you are the best lover ever.

"It's particularly important for women to have successful foreplay because it takes a woman a longer time [than a man] to get up to the level of arousal needed to orgasm," says "Dr. Ruth" Westheimer, EdD, a psychosexual therapist, professor at New York University, and lecturer at Yale and Princeton universities.

Foreplay starts with things like listening, eye contact, opening building doors and car doors, pulling out her chair, holding her hand, touching her softly, unexpected flowers, and breakfast in bed, making her favorite dinner, surprising her with her favorite perfume, the list could go on and on.

It culminates with the pre-sexual cursor of touch, smell, sight and tease. None of the techniques are difficult to implement, if you love your partner, make her think she is special and unique to you. These gentlemen like gestures should continue for the duration of a relationship, not just at the beginning.

The Art of Making a Woman Relax

Most women will not feel "in the mood" for sex if they are not relaxed. That makes it important to know what ways your partner relaxes and what measures you can take to help her relax.

For women to get in the mood for sexual activity, internal and external stresses need to be shut down, and when we help shut this down, women feel like we've contributed to their feeling of relaxation.

The following techniques could work for different women to help them relax:

- A neck or back massage;
- A foot massage;
- A bath;
- Relaxing with her in a hot tub will do the trick.
- Stroking her hair while she listens to her favorite CD.

You need to figure that out with your partner. Every relationship is different.

The five senses (touch, smell, sight, taste, and hearing) also play a role in putting her mind at ease. A woman's body will not get excited unless her mind is at ease. If her mind is at ease, her body will be at ease, and her body will be in a wonderful place for excitement.

The Five Senses

We've briefly touched on the roe the sense can play in all of this, the following pages describe the senses individually.

Sight

Aside from physical attraction, sight can also be important based on the cleanliness of the surroundings the sexual intercourse is about to take place in. Therefore, it's important to keep the room (more often than not the bedroom) tidy and make your partner feel at ease and comfortable.

Women will appreciate it if you clean your sheets, pick up the underwear, and remove the dishes that are beginning to collect flies and mold. Make her feel like you have some respect for yourself.

Hearing

Women respond well to seduction through their ears. Complimenting her softly directly into her ear is a great way to get them excited.

In the same way, external noises such as an instrumental cd in the background can heighten the mood. It's generally better to play music without lyrics to remove awkward lyrics and the temptation to concentrate on the lyrics and to really soothe the mind.

Taste

Food and drink can also play a part in the entire sexual experience, with some foods making excellent and romantic props in the bedroom. A few foods to try are olives, strawberries, grapes, chocolate or cheese. Wine is a nice alcohol that goes well with cheese and chocolate. A clean mouth is always a must, which all of you know.

Smell

The section of the brain that registers smells and recall scents plays a powerful role in seduction, and it's the reason perfume sells so well. We associate smells with people or places, so it's important to create a similar feeling and memory triggers for romance and sex with you and your partner.

Women can be turned on strongly by a man's cologne, or even natural scent. But it's also a good idea to keep a flavored candle burning or plug in an air freshener as well to give the area a nice smell.

Touch

Once you have done your best to relax her other 4 senses, now it is time to relax her body with your touch.

Women respond best to touch, and will be all yours if you're listening to her body and focusing on her movements to understand what she wants. You will notice her breathing getting faster or deeper.

How to Relax her Body

Now that you have learned how to relax her mind, it is time for you to learn how to relax her body

The aim of relaxing her body is to make her feel like there's no other place in the world that you would want to be. Long kisses, touches, eye contact and teasing are all part of this process and all contribute to the total relaxation of the mind and the culmination of successful foreplay.

Strictly speaking, women don't necessarily need to be touched sexually to become aroused or relaxed. Many women prefer just to be hugged, held, or kissed on the forehead by the man they were with. It makes them feel wanted and loved, which in turn opens them up sexually.

Kissing is the romantic gesture that ignites most sexual encounters and often gets a woman in the mood more than any other method. Kissing can vary from quick pecks, to long lasting kisses, all work well to build romanticism and create eroticism. Women respond different to different kissing styles so make sure you know what your woman likes and at the different times she wants them.

Spontaneity is your friend in the art of kissing. Try stealing a moment by grabbing her by the arm and kissing her when she is brushing her hair or cleaning up her dishes. Kiss her against the wall, holding her hands to her side, or cradling the sides of her head in your hands. This will begin the buildup to sexual excitement.

The art of foreplay is getting her entire body ready for sex, don't miss any part of her body. Touch her face, head, neck, ears, feet, legs, back, breasts, stomach, buttocks, shoulders, hands, and vagina with your kisses and touches. Massage those areas in the way she likes it, either hard of soft, oily or dry.

The following techniques associated with touch should work wonders with your partner (individual preferences aside):

- The shoulders and neck are a very sensitive area for women and an area that if touched properly can get them truly aroused. Use your lips, fingers and tongue in nice circular motions with very light pressure.

- A sweet spot on all women is from the bottom of her ear to the top of her neck. Sweep away her hair and slowly kiss and lick her neck down to her shoulders.

- The back can withstand a slightly heavier touch and is therefore a great area for deeper touches and massages. The sacral curve, located above the curve of her buttocks, is a sensitive area on a women's back and can bring great excitement to her when rubbed and touched. Rubbing the lower back and buttocks can stimulate the groin area.

- Casting a woman's doubts about showing her bottom to you, this again can provide an excellent platform for excitement and experimentation. Only you and your partner can determine how comfortable you both are with this area, but it does allow for some sexy scenarios and discovery.

- The breasts, often the man's favorite spot, should only be touched sparingly. While they are sensitive and do add to the sexual experience, too much time is often spent gravitating to these areas and losing focus on other areas like the ones above. It's best to touch and lick these carefully and conservatively.

- Hair is another area that women love having touched and played with. To do so effectively, massage the upper portion of the neck and lift up the hair and kiss your partner for the ultimate turn on. A nice scalp rub, or the feeling of hot breath against their head will also make a woman excited.

- The face is made up of more elements that add to the sec and foreplay experience. It's important to be gentle on the face as it's made up of the lips, jaw, nose and other sensitive parts that are also important for bodily functions. Use the tips of your fingers and tongue to trace the outline of the features.

- Penultimately, try focusing some attention on the ears and ear lobes. Along with playful attention of the ears try breathing lightly in her ear so she knows you're there and can respond to your advances.

- Lastly, the limbs (feet, hands, wrists and arms) are an area to focus the touch on throughout the day. Because they can be touched in public they helped create a buildup of the sexual tension as well as help create intimacy in a relationship. Not only that the touch of the limbs could cure ailments and reduce tension.

The major lesson to take out of this all and the foreplay and relaxation advice given above, is that it's important to understand your partners body and her needs and wants. Be patient and open to communication with your partner and as you learn more about her, your sexual endeavors will be far more fruitful.

By focusing on mutual foreplay and not about "getting off" will shift your attention from you to her, and in turn keep your mind off the importance of lasting longer in bed. The mind is very, very powerful so this report recommends using it to its full potential to help overcome your sexual anxiety.

A More Intimate Touch

As explained during the explanation of touch above, fingers play an important part in discover a partner's body and discovering what she likes. The same can be said with the fingers during foreplay, especially when in contact with the vagina. Communication is the key once more to understand how your partner likes to be touched.

Start with clean hands, with trimmed nails and always was your hands thoroughly before coming into contact with a lady's sensitive areas.

To build up sexual excitement, some women will like immediate clitoral stimulation, whereas others may prefer warming up in other areas such as the vulva. We recommend using lubricant, to prevent the women from drying out and add to the excitement levels. It can be exciting finding a lubricant that works for you. This could include flavored, oil based or water based, and experimentation is half the fun.

Women will usually guide you in this approach by moving their torso in the direction they want you to stimulate. Follow their movements to find a spot that they are happy with.

Regardless of what move or position you are in when you are using your fingers on her, it is important to start with bigger motions and then moving to smaller more concentrated motions. You also want to slowly build your speed. Start off slowly and gradually start moving faster.

Here's a full-proof method that this report recommends:

1. It is easy to find out what will make your lady most excited by varying tempo, degree of pressure, and the motion of your fingers. It is always a good idea to rest the palm of your hand on the area where the pubic hair starts (mons pubis) and apply pressure. Place a well lubricated hand over her labia, fingers pointing towards her anus. Pull up toward the navel. Experiment by touching her inner and outer lips gently. Pull softly on one lip and then the other. Rub the outer lips gently between your forefinger and thumb, then the inner lips.

2. Place the palm of your hand on her pubic hair region and rest your fingers lightly on her lips. Put your thumb on her thigh. Gently, but with pressure, press your palm onto her mons pubis and begin to move your hand in a small circular motion. Your palm should not move too much over her skin during this process. Instead, her skin should move underneath your palm.

3. Repeat this process until you have done 8-10 circles. You will then raise your fingers and softly tap her vaginal lips about once every second until you have given her 8-10 taps. After you have done this, rest your hand for 6-8 seconds. Then repeat the whole routine over as much as you and your partner fancy.

Conclusion

This report has been compiled to help you last longer at sex, but deeper than that it could also help in your overall sexual performance and the foundation of your relationship through intimacy and communication. Start some of the exercises today and be patient and confident that if you follow them as we've explained them here, that you will be well on your way to sexual success and fulfillment.

Good Luck!

Learn More

Visit MensGrowth.com to check out the latest advice for men who are looking to be ambitious... Master their lifestyle... Perform in the bedroom... Experience better health, wealth and personal growth...

www.MensGrowth.com

Newsletter

Sign up to MensGrowth.com newsletter to get strategies for better health, increased wealth, style, sex and personal growth news to your inbox. **www.MensGrowth.com/join**